What Is Homeopathy?

Vinton McCabe

A Basic Health Guide

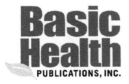

The information contained in this book is based upon the research and personal and professional experiences of the author. It is not intended as a substitute for consulting with your physician or other healthcare provider. Any attempt to diagnose and treat an illness should be done under the direction of a healthcare professional.

The publisher does not advocate the use of any particular healthcare protocol but believes the information in this book should be available to the public. The publisher and author are not responsible for any adverse effects or consequences resulting from the use of the suggestions, preparations, or procedures discussed in this book. Should the reader have any questions concerning the appropriateness of any procedures or preparation mentioned, the author and the publisher strongly suggest consulting a professional healthcare advisor.

Basic Health Publications, Inc.
www.basichealthpub.com

Library of Congress Cataloging-in-Publication Data

Library of Congress Cataloging-in-Publication Data is available through the Library of Congress.

ISBN 978-1-59120-297-4 (Pbk.)
ISBN 978-1-68162-912-4 (Hardcover)

Editor: Karen Anspach
Typesetting/Book design: Gary A. Rosenberg
Cover design: Mike Stromberg

Contents

About the Author

Vinton McCabe has studied homeopathy for the past thirty years, and has been a homeopathic educator, activist and author for the past quarter of a century. He is the author of nine books on the subject of health and healing, including his latest book, *What is Homeopathy?*, a consideration of the Bach Flower Remedies called *The Healing Bouquet*, and the now-standard text *Practical Homeopathy*. He is also the author of the Kindle-exclusive line of e-books in the "Homeopathy in Thought & Action" series and is the author/creator of the popular blog *Psora Psora Psora*.

In addition, McCabe has served on the faculty of the Connecticut Homeopathic Association, the Open Center in Manhattan and the Wainwright House in Rye, New York as a homeopathic educator. He has also taught homeopathy at the Learning Annex, the Omega Institute, the New York Botanical Garden and the Seminar Center in Manhattan. He has appeared nationally as an advocate for homeopathic health care on such programs as "The Gary Null Show."

As a print journalist, Vinton McCabe has worked for publications, including *New England Monthly*, *The Stamford Advocate*, and *The New York Times*. He served as Arts Editor both for the *Advocate* newspapers of Connecticut and Massachusetts and for *Corpus Christi Magazine* in Texas.

He lives in Litchfield County, Connecticut and, aside from his work in homeopathy, McCabe now works as a book reviewer for the New York Journal of Books.

For more information on homeopathy,
please visit my website:
www.vintonmccabe.com

What is Homeopathy?

To understand the word "homeopathy," you have to go back two hundred years. To understand the concept of homeopathy, you have to go back two thousand.

But to understand the *need* for homeopathy in the world today, you only have to open your eyes, both to the world around you and those who populate it—their needs, their chronic aches and pains as well as their acute day-to-day needs—and to yourself. Take a look at yourself in the mirror, a good, long look. Do you like what you see? Are you satisfied with your state of health, or do you think that it could be improved?

In general, I have always had an issue with the term "alternative medicine," because I think that in accepting the word *alternative*, those of us who consider homeopathy to be our primary form of medical treatment agree to allow our beliefs to be defined not by what homeopathy is and what it has to offer, but instead by our culture's primary form of medical treatment: allopathy. As someone who has made his living with words and in the communication of ideas, I can't help but recognize that, in yielding the status quo to allopathic medicine, homeopathy marginalizes itself and forces itself into a niche.

However, the more I watch TV and read newspapers and Internet reports of court cases and clinical trials that prove again and again just how dangerous allopathic drugs can be and how toxic allopathic medicine is in both philosophy and practice, the more I read of drugs like those for the treatment of diabetes that, in treating diabetes cause heart attacks, the more willing I become to embrace the word *alternative*.

Because homeopathic medicine offers each of us a true alternative to the dangers of "traditional" allopathic medicine. An alternative that is both effective and safe. And given that allopathic medicine is neither of these, that is a pretty potent promise.

And yet, it is not the purpose of this text to simply damn allopathic medicine. Nor is it my purpose to limit the choice of any consumer when it comes to the selection of an appropriate form of medical treatment. Instead, the purpose of this book is to inform and educate the reader not just about homeopathy, but about medicine in general, and especially to educate on the subject of healing and how it most easily and reliably can be achieved, no matter the illness or its cause.

A Medical Truism, with Apologies to Abraham Lincoln

When you are thinking about *any* form of medicine, consider this: *All medicine can cure some of the people all of the time and all of the people some of the time. But no medicine can cure all the people all of the time.*

You need to remember this, because it is true. Any form of medicine will work for any patient sometimes, under conditions that are ideal for that medical modality. For the patient with a stiff neck, for instance, chiropractic medicine can work wonders, where it may not work as well for the patient with heart disease. This is not to say that chiropractic medicine has no value, only that, like everything else, it does not represent a cure-all. Nothing does. Allopathic medicine may work well for a given patient in many instances in his or her life—it is, for instance, very good in medical emergencies—but it may utterly fail under other circumstances. The same may be said about homeopathic medicine or Traditional Chinese Medicine or Ayurvada or anything else.

This is partially true due to the differing skill levels of the practitioners of any form of medicine. The perfectly good allopath trained in family medicine may not have the skill set required for a patient who presents symptoms with which he is unfamiliar. And that patient may then be sent through the full maze of allopathic tests, probes, and specialists, all without result. In the same way, the homeopath who is wonderfully skilled at treating constitutionally may not make the right decision in terms of a remedy when faced with a sudden acute ailment requiring an immediate decision that does not allow the practitioner to make full use of his or her many different Materia Medicas, Repertories, and computer software packages.

But I think that my bastardization of Lincoln's truism goes beyond the practitioners to the medical modalities themselves. I believe that no form of medicine will ever be a cure-all for all patients at all times, no matter how skilled the practitioners of all these various forms of medicine may be. The various modalities of medicine work with the body in different ways, exacting different costs and offering different benefits. Therefore, I think it wise for patients to become wise consumers of *all* forms of medicine and to know the appropriate use of each—and before advocates of natural medicine close this book, let me hasten to point out that herbal medicine is, by its very nature, allopathic, so let's throw into this discussion the fact that many of these different forms of medicine have good and bad aspects as well. All the forms of medicine mentioned here—and let's add acupuncture, healing hands, and nutritional/naturopathic medicine into the mix—have been shown effective in both clinical trials and in the lives of individual patients over not just decades but over millennia. It is therefore the purpose of this book to throw no babies out with their various tubs of bathwater. I do not seek to inhibit the use of any form of medicine, only to explain the why and how of homeopathy and to give the reader an understanding of the reasons why it belongs, right next to allopathy, at the top of the list of potential treatments that are readily available to *all* wise consumers of medicine.

CHAPTER 1

Definitions

In beginning a study of homeopathy, we have to first consider the meaning of a few key terms, words that we use often enough that we all assume that we are in agreement about their meaning. And yet it is important that we all know what we are talking about when we use them:

Medicine

All branches of medicine come from the same source materials. All medicine began with herbal and other natural substances. And all forms of medical philosophy are based upon direct experience with the animal, vegetable, or mineral substance used for a medicinal purpose. Substances are considered "medicinal" for the simple reason that they can create a more-or-less predictable change in the human system. Ancient man found that ingesting a root or a leaf could cause nausea or alleviate nausea; that the application of a leaf directly to the skin could soothe a wound. Thus it is the basic fact that the substance can create a *change* that makes it medicinal and that fact that the change is more often *predictable* than it is not that makes the substance useful as a medicine. But note that the change created can be for good or ill— that the situation at hand often determines whether a substance can be considered a medicine or a toxin. What may be helpful to one patient may be harmful to another. It is also important to note that, when I use the word *change*, I should actually be using the plural *changes*. No medicine, as we shall see, does only one thing, all bring about a number of changes at once, some more predictable than others. Some systems of medical practice take into account all the changes that a particular medicine brings about, others do not, as we shall see. But all medicines work by creating what can be considered a series of *artificial symptoms* that, when the medicine is taken, have an impact on the natural symptoms already in place. Think about it: if you were to take an over-the-counter cold medicine when you did not have any symptoms of a cold, what would the cold medicine do? How would it make you feel? What changes could you expect to take place from taking it? It is because a medicine can artificially create (inflict) a number of symptoms (changes) in the human system that it is useful. Therefore, the science of medicine, at its heart, is a system of inquiry and treatment that seeks to match the symptoms at hand with the best option (in terms of a specific medicine that creates a known set of artificial symptoms) to use to alleviate a given disease. Different forms of medicine take different approaches as to how this should be done.

Curing

Most forms of medicine speak of curing diseases. But what is meant by that? What does the word *cure* actually mean? The implication is that, in curing a disease, an external force acts upon a given symptom or set of symptoms with the result of removing them. But does this, in fact, ever take place? Does such a thing as a cure exist? Think of that cold medicine again. When you are ill and you take an over-the-counter cold medicine, does that medicine in any way affect the actual cold that you are experiencing, or does it instead merely inhibit your ability to experience the cold symptoms that you have? And, more important, does that cold medicine in any way strengthen your system so that you are less likely to get another cold in the future? After all, every form of medicine depends upon your body's ability to heal itself in order to set things right. Some medicine, as we shall see, works by suppressing symptoms in a waiting game. Others work by strengthening your own natural ability to heal, but still depend upon the body's own ability. Indeed, even the surgeon who heroically operates on a patient's heart and repairs damage done to it still depends upon the fact that that patient's body can heal itself of the trauma of the surgery. The more you think about it, the more I think you will come to share my conclusion—that there is no such thing as curing a disease. A medical practitioner can intervene to create circumstances in which the healing process can be assisted or inhibited, but a doctor, in fact, has no power to cure anything.

Healing

Where curing is an external thing—an external force impacting the patient's body, mind, and spirit through the use of some medicine—healing is both an internal and a natural thing. Many methods of attempting to cure diseases are far from natural, but the healing process is inborn. We humans have an innate ability to heal. In my opinion, we have a nearly limitless ability to heal, if that ability is given free reign. The best treatments, therefore, are those that strengthen and encourage this natural process—that work *with* the body's own healing talent. The wise physician, therefore, studies not just disease but also health and, especially, the healing process. The best practitioner is one who has studied how healing takes place and how it can be encouraged, and how a patient's own natural immunity can be maintained in the long term, so that it is both balanced and strong.

Sickness & Health

The Greek homeopath George Vithoulkas refers to healing simply as "the restoration of happiness." In this brief definition, he suggests that healing involves the spiritual as well as the physical plane. Samuel Hahnemann, the Father of Homeopathy writes, in the first paragraph of his book *The Organon of the Healing Art*: "The physician's high and only mission is to restore the sick to health...." But what does he mean by this? We tend to oversimplify our definitions when it comes to health and healing, and to look at the situation as if there were a switch that could be turned off and on. One day we are healthy. The next we are sick. In reality, there is a continuum of sickness and health and each of us lives our lives somewhere within that continuum. For most of us, even when we consider ourselves to be "healthy," that is only a relative term. Even on our best days we have weaknesses and aches and pains. Some few live on the high end of the continuum and are what may be considered truly healthy. And unfortunate millions live at the opposite end of the spectrum and live lives in which they are besieged by one ailment after another. (Because of this, their definition of health might well be what a truly healthy person would still think of as being sick. Health, sickness, and healing are all, truthfully, relative terms.) The majority of us live in the middle of the continuum—while we have some degree of health, we also tend to always have some joint pain, acid reflux, or sleep issues. When it comes to defining health and sickness, for me they both come down to a single concept, and that concept is *freedom*. The extent to which we may live our individual lives in a state of freedom of movement, of positive thought and mood and intent is the extent to which we may consider ourselves to be healthy. And the more restricted we are—by our bodies, by our emotions, and/or by our thoughts—the less healthy we are, because we are less free to live a life without restriction. Those with chronic diseases of any sort are aware that the life lived within boundaries imposed by a disease state are lives that, over time, come to be more or less defined by the disease and not by the visions or goals that the healthy are free to set for themselves.

Doctors & Physicians

The term *doctor* refers to a medical degree and a medical license. It is an honorific that most practitioners feel is earned by hard work and dedication. While I in no way denigrate the term, I do want to point out that the word physician, which is often used interchangeably with the word doctor, means something quite different. *Physician* comes from the Greek word *physis*, which was coined by Hippocrates, the Father of Medicine. It was the term he gave for the body's own natural healing process. Therefore, a physician is technically a person who works with the healing process and encourages it in order for the sick to be made well. *Physician* does not imply a degree or a license; instead, it implies a method of thought and action—one that is in accordance with natural law. It is, therefore, sometimes possible to find a doctor who is a physician as well, but it is also likely in many cases that the two terms may be mutually exclusive.

In closing this chapter, I ask that you take a moment and consider the following:

- *Can you be healed without being cured?* In what ways might this be possible?

- *Can you be cured without being healed?* In what ways might this be possible?

In time, and with some consideration of the concepts presented and the questions posed, you will find your own set of answers to the riddle of health and healing. Indeed, the best answers are the ones that you discover for yourself, as you wrestle with your own health and the health of those that you love. There is no one best answer for every person, as my warped version of Abraham Lincoln's quote suggests.

But in learning the difference between curing and healing, doctors and physicians and sickness and health, we can better come to understand the nature of medicine itself, and, in doing so, can find the method or methods of treatment that will grant us access to those two words that best sum up the state of being that can be called healthy: freedom and happiness.

With these basic definitions in place, let us next consider the primary differences between the two most basic methods of treatment, the homeopathic and the allopathic.

CHAPTER 2

Homeopathy and Allopathy

When we get down to basics, all medicine falls into one or the other of two categories: allopathic or homeopathic. This includes *all* medicine, from Traditional Chinese Medicine—which contains components that are homeopathic in nature and others that are allopathic—to herbal medicine, which, although natural, is allopathic.

The difference between the two categories has to do with a patient's symptoms—and how these symptoms are considered and how they are treated.

Indeed, the words "homeopathy" and "allopathy" themselves describe each modality's philosophy and how a practitioner in each field of medicine will treat the symptoms of any given illness:

Homeopathy comes from two Greek words: homios, meaning "similar" and pathos, meaning "suffering." The term homeopathy, as coined by Samuel Hahnemann (1755-1843) a couple hundred years ago, literally means "similar suffering." The word itself, therefore, references the central concept of homeopathic treatment, the principle of "Similars" or Similarity, as we shall refer to it here, which, simply stated, is "like cures like." By this I mean that, when a patient goes to see a homeopathic physician, that patient will be given a remedy that works with his symptoms and not against them. He will be given a remedy that, in a totally well person, would artificially create the same symptoms that the patient is experiencing naturally. In Hahnemann's day, these were revolutionary thoughts, and Hahnemann, in insisting upon them, created a stir in the medical world similar to that which Martin Luther created in the world of religion. With the coining of the term homeopathy, a new school of medical practice was born.

Allopathy is another medical term coined by Samuel Hahnemann to describe what he called the "old school" of medicine, the one that he was rebelling against because he found that, in his medical practice, more patients were dying from their toxic medicines than were dying of their diseases. The word allopathy is also taken from two Greek words: *allos*, meaning "different," and pathos once again as the suffix. Allopathy, therefore, literally means "different suffering." And allopathic treatments follow the same philosophy. If a patient with a given set of symptoms goes to see an allopathic doctor, he is given a drug whose action is to artificially create a set of symptoms that are in opposition to those that the patient is already experiencing. If the patient has a runny nose, for instance, he will be given a substance that will cause his nose to dry up and stop running.

The differing opinion as to how symptoms should be treated is the most basic difference between allopathic and homeopathic medicine. And, because we were all raised in an allopathic culture, the idea of working *with* symptoms, actually enhancing them, will likely strike you as odd at first, but let's consider some other ways that homeopathic medicine differs from allopathic.

Before we discuss these differences, I want to put an image in your mind, one originally described by Hippocrates, the first physician we know of (much of the history of medicine is lost in the mist of time) who elaborated on the principles that would one day be named homeopathic and allopathic.

Hippocrates described the two methods of treatment as being twin streams that flowed side by side. They looked exactly alike and they lay in riverbeds that were exactly parallel to each other from start to finish, so they never touched, never connected. The difference between these two clear, cool streams of flowing water was that they flowed in opposite directions. No medicine can be both homeopathic and allopathic at the same time. Their impact upon the body is in direct opposition to each other: one suppressing symptoms, as we shall see, and driving symptoms deeper into the body, the other expressing them and removing them from the body.

With this in mind, let's consider some other key differences between homeopathy and allopathy.

Symptoms

While I have already stated that these two systems of medical treatment differ in the way they treat symptoms, it's important to mention exactly why, as homeopathic and allopathic medicine define the concept of symptoms differently. In allopathic medicine, symptoms are seen in a quasi-militaristic way. Symptoms are seen as invaders, usually germs, that sneak into our bodies when someone sneezes or shakes our hand. Once inside our bodies, the germs grow and fester and cause us all sorts of trouble. Symptoms are therefore things that move from the outside world into our bodies. They are bad and must be eliminated at all costs.

And, perhaps most important, the allopathic model of medicine sees the patient as being in a state of health when the symptoms are eliminated, as if health is lurking below the surface, ready to spring forth again if and when the invading symptoms are eliminated.

In homeopathic medicine, symptoms are seen in a different light. They are considered to be good things. In the first place, they are the sign that the immune system is working. It has kicked in to combat some threat, a virus or bacteria perhaps, that has been identified in the body. Symptoms are seen in homeopathic medicine as reactive things, not invaders. When the immune system identifies a threat, it attempts to balance the body by creating a fever, or by flooding the system with mucus. The fever and the mucus, therefore, are not seen as something that is bad, but as a sign that the body is functioning exactly as it should. For this reason, the homeopath's task is to help the body do the work that it is already doing, but to do it more swiftly, more safely, and more effectively. It is, therefore, never the role of the homeopathic physician to try and cure anything. Instead, he seeks to try to assist the patient's body as it heals itself, using homeopathic remedies to assist the immune factor (or the Vital Force as it is sometimes called in homeopathic medicine) in expressing or pushing outward the symptoms of disease and, in doing so, restoring the patient to a state of health. The homeopathic physician will also, through studying the specific symptoms displayed by the patient, work with the patient's own unique nature, tailoring his treatment to that patient alone. The manifestation of a specific set of symptoms will point the homeopath to the specific remedy needed to bring about the best possible result.

This is one of the chief differences between homeopathy and allopathy. The allopath uses the diagnosis of a particular disease, from the common cold to cancer, as more or less a road map of the treatment that will then be given. He will have a set group of medicines that are called upon to combat that disease and will choose from those medicines the one (or more) that he feels will work best to treat the disease at hand.

The homeopath, on the other hand, will never make an assumption of what medicine will be most effective based upon the diagnosis of the disease alone. It is always the goal of homeopathic treatment to match the remedy in the full sphere of its actions with the patient in the full range of his symptoms. The homeopath will then choose the medicine that he thinks will best serve the patient. In other words, when beginning the process of homeopathic treatment, the disease diagnosis does not present a fixed map for treatment. Treatment is based upon the needs of the patient and not upon the most commonly used medicines for the disease.

One of the great mistakes that allopaths make is to systematize their medicine—to make the assumption that all patients with the same diseases will be more or less the same in terms of their response to treatment and the mere presence of a specific disease can suggest a specific form of treatment. This, along with their willingness to believe that they can separate the desired effect of a given medicine from its "side effects" and their belief in *polypharmacy* (giving one, two, three, or more medicines at the same time) is why allopathic medicine is as toxic today as it was in Hahnemann's day.

Uniquity and Wholeness

Together, these two concepts reach the heart of homeopathic philosophy. Just as homeopaths and allopaths differ as to what symptoms are and how they should be treated, they also differ on the nature of the patient himself and the ways in which medicine can be used.

It is very important that we understand why, in homeopathic medicine, the patient is seen as both a *unique* and a *whole* being. It was American homeopath James Tyler Kent who first stated that the best-prepared homeopathic remedy *ceases to be homeopathic if it is used with allopathic methods*. This means that if we start using homeopathic remedies without first understanding homeopathic philosophy, we can never use them correctly. By understanding both the concepts of *uniquity* and *wholeness*, we better prepare ourselves to adhere to the methods of homeopathic healing.

• **Uniquity:** When entering a homeopath's office for the first time, be prepared to answer questions that may seem a bit odd at first—questions like how thirsty you are, what food cravings and aversions you might have, what your common sleep positions are, etc. These questions will be asked in addition to the standard questions about your reason for your visit, of course—the ailment that brought you into the office in the first place. But even the questions asked about the symptoms of your illness may seem strange. It will, for instance, be important to the homeopath whether your sore throat started on the left side of your throat or the right. Or whether your illness came on quickly or developed slowly. The homeopath asks these questions as well as examines you to learn as much about you as possible—to identify all the things about you that make you unique. Because, to a homeopath, we are all unique beings. The ways in which you remain healthy or become ill may or may not have anything to do with the ways in which anyone else does. And the ways in which you express an illness—the symptoms—may be very different from the ways in which I express the same illness. Two patients with the same cold in the same season—an illness caused by the same set of circumstances—may well need different homeopathic treatments. The treatment must always be geared to the patient, not the disease. Why? Because we are all completely unique beings. To make the mistake of basing the treatment on the *disease* is to treat the patient allopathically, no matter what kind of pill—homeopathic or allopathic—is given.

• **Wholeness:** Along this same line of thinking, homeopathic medicine also upholds the concept of *wholeness*. Allopathic medicine has, over the last few centuries, managed to divide us into many parts, many organs and systems of organs. They have also managed to reduce everything, from our sexual urges to our thought processes, down to chemical reactions. Adherents to homeopathic medicine disagree. To the homeopath, you are one whole being and *no two symptoms can ever be anything other than connected in a whole being*. Therefore, when you are treated by a homeopath, *all* your symptoms must be considered. If your head hurts on the right side at 4:00 P.M. and your legs twitch in bed at night, then both of these symptoms, as well as their unique timing, must be considered, and considered as being of equal import in deciding upon a homeopathic treatment.

Therefore, we will never see a homeopathic "specialist"—a homeopathic heart specialist or homeopathic allergist. Homeopathy rejects the concept of specialists; the homeopath always looks at the whole person. A being of body, mind, and spirit, in which all three are at all times interrelated.

And so, when you are treated by a homeopath, you are treated as a unique and whole being. Almost a universe unto yourself with your own laws of harmony and disharmony. It is the job of the homeopath to try to discover the appropriate treatment so that the patient's whole being can be brought into balance. The result is that the patient improves not only in terms of the ailment that brought him into the office in the first place; he is also left in a healthier state in general. The homeopath not only seeks to help the patient with his headache, he also seeks to prevent the patient from having another headache in the future.

This is only possible if the treatment is geared not to the headache, but to the patient and his own unique needs.

The other great mistake that the allopath makes is his belief that his medical treatments can impact just one part of the body and leave the rest untouched. We are whole beings, interconnected in body, mind, and spirit. That which touches one part of us touches all. The

allopath, once again, chalks the myriad changes—some dangerous—
that his medicines create to just being "side effects." And while the
allopath is usually all too willing to accept these side effects as necessary evils, the side effects are often the toxic reality of allopathic treatments for the patient. Far from being the little inconveniences that
the term implies, side effects can be dangerous and are as much a part of
the action of any allopathic drug as is the primary action for which the
drug is used.

Side Effects

Just a couple more thoughts on this topic before we move on.

If you want to see what I am talking about in terms of the allopathic concept of the primary action of a remedy versus the side
effects, take a look in any *Physician's Desk Reference*. This large book
will be in the office of any allopathic doctor. Look up any drug you
like, for any disease: hypertension, diabetes, lupus—it doesn't matter.
The listing is always the same. First discussed is the "primary action,"
which is to say the desired action, the reason why the drug is used.
This tells you what, in clinical experience, the drug has been seen
capable of doing, what changes it can more or less predictably make in
the human system.

What follows then is a list of side effects. There may be paragraphs
of them, or there may literally be pages and pages. The allopathic medical model seeks to divide the primary action of the drug—the "good"
that the drug does, from its side effects—the "bad" things that the drug
also does, and to pretend that the trade-off is worth it. Further, when
the drug is studied and used, it is used based upon the primary action,
and not the side effects. The side effects are usually only considered
when they begin to manifest through the use of the drug.

The simple reality is that—and this is vitally important, so
remember it—no medicine does only one thing. All medicines have
many different actions in the human system. And these actions can
impact upon all three parts of the whole being—the body, the mind,
and the spirit/emotions. For this reason medicines of all sorts—homeopathic and allopathic—must be studied and understood in the full

sphere of their activities, for all the myriad changes they can potentially cause in the human system, and not be given based on the false
hope that the good will outweigh the bad.

In homeopathic medicine, there are no such things as side effects.
Not because homeopathic medicines miraculously do only one thing,
have only one impact on the human system. They have no side effects
because, when a homeopathic remedy is tested and proven in its
actions,, its full range of impact is noted before it is added to the
homeopathic pharmacy. Homeopathic remedies are the only medicines that are tested on healthy human beings. Allopathic medicines
are tested either on animals or on sick patients. Homeopathic remedies are tested in double-blind studies in which the remedy is taken
repeatedly and each and every change experienced by the test group is
noted. Comparisons are then made among the findings of the whole
group given the potent remedy (as opposed to the test group given the
placebo) and all potential impact of the remedy is noted and studied.

Therefore, when a homeopathic remedy is given, it is given
because its totality of action best matches the totality of the patient's
symptoms. Because all the actions of the remedy are fully taken into
account, no remedy is ever given with the allopathic illusion that one
aspect of the medicine's impact can be separated out from the rest, and
the rest can be assigned the benign name "side effects," and that they
will be little things of no real importance.

Homeopathic treatments take into account the full range of
actions that a given remedy creates. It works by matching the totality
of a remedy's actions to the totality of a patient's symptoms. For this
reason homeopathic treatments are far safer than allopathic treatments. And because homeopathic treatments take into account the
many actions of a given remedy, they also are most often given as single medicines and are not used in conjunction with two, three, or
more other medicines in order to "get the job done." This makes
homeopathic treatments far safer and far more predictable in terms of
restoring patients to a state of health.

CHAPTER 3

What Homeopathy Does *Not* Treat

I get asked this question all the time. What is homeopathy *good for*? And what does homeopathy *not* treat?

The simple answer is that homeopathy is a fully developed medical modality, capable of treating anything that standard Western (allopathic) medicine can treat, and that homeopathy can offer treatments that are at once cheaper, safer, and more effective than allopathic treatments. But more on that last part later.

The more complicated answer to the same question can sound, on first hearing it, as if I am trying to dodge the question altogether.

The answer is that the one thing that homeopathy does *not* treat is disease. Homeopathic medicine is never used in the treatment of any disease. It is, instead, used to treat patients who *have* various ailments and diseases.

This can sound like a coy answer to an important question, but the distinction between treating a disease and a patient with a disease is huge, and an understanding of this distinction is hugely important.

It can also be hard to grasp. Even students who have just taken a class on the philosophy and practice of homeopathy have been known to walk up to me after the class and tell me that they have a backache and ask what remedy they should take.

Even after having listened and taken notes, they seem surprised when I end up shaking my head and saying, "It doesn't work that way."

Admittedly, it is a hard concept to grasp. The vast majority of us have, for so long now, lived with the medical concept that, if I have this pain I take that pill. So when someone comes along and says that this idea is not only wrong but actually ineffective in the long run and possibly dangerous, the shift in thinking takes some getting used to. And certainly our pill-centric culture, in which many pills are brightly colored or colorfully coated to look as much like candy as possible, is partially to blame. Our media is filled with advertising that not only promises that this bleach will get our clothes whiter, but also that this pill or that liquid will allow us to *not* experience our cold or allergy symptoms—to pretend that we are not sick—for an extended period of time.

We have been raised on a lot of myths when it comes to medicine. That pills are most often the solution. ("Why don't you just go to the doctor and get some pills?") That medicine works by virtue of quid pro quo—you have this, you take that and, bingo, all better. That taking medicine is a natural thing, a good thing—that it is so natural and good that we should also give our pets medications on a regular basis and buy them health insurance while we are at it.

The greatest myth is that, when it comes to medicine, one size fits all. That all people with a cold will benefit from the same treatment. That any disease can act as a map for the best possible treatment. This would work just fine if we were all the same—if we had the same genes, the same characteristics, the same thought processes. But the myth that a population as diverse as the human race can all respond equally well to the same form of treatment seems beyond foolish. It seems (to me at least) to belong to the same childhood belief system as making a wish while we blow out the candles on a birthday cake or trying to stay up late to catch Santa sneaking down the chimney.

When I say that homeopathy does not treat diseases, but, instead, treats patients with diseases, I am trying to dispel some myths: That medicine is easy. That diseases can be cured or managed or in any way controlled. That by naming something, we can control it.

The reality is that the human being remains largely a mysterious thing, in body, mind, and spirit. And that what medical science knows about the human being is still dwarfed by what medical science does not know.

Homeopathic medicine seeks to take another approach. In doing so, its philosophy and practice differs from allopathic medicine in some ways that I truly appreciate. First, it is always the goal of homeopathic treatment to get the patient off medication as soon as possible. Homeopathic remedies are not meant to be taken continually as a means of "managing" a disease. Instead, they are given in order to stimulate the patient's ability to heal himself, and, once healed, the patient no longer needs to continue to take the remedy.

Another way homeopathy is different is this whole idea of treating the patient as a whole and unique being. But how does this work?

Take that student of mine who had the backache. The allopath would give him a painkiller, possibly an anti-inflammatory and send him on his way, with advice about alternating hot and cold, or just applying heat, depending upon the situation. The homeopath would first consider the nature of the backache. Is it a simple acute situation, caused by a mechanical injury or by being forced to sit in an uncomfortable chair as I yammer on and on at the front of the room? Or is it something more, something deeper—is this backache one of many that the student has experienced over a period of time? The homeopath always first tries to grasp the reason for the onset of the disease, if possible, and always questions the patient's susceptibility to a given condition.

Indeed, my bastardized Lincoln quote can be used for illness as well as medicine: *All illness can kill some of the people all of the time and all of the people some of the time, but no illness can kill all of the people all of the time.*

Why? Because of the concept of *susceptibility*. No matter how new or violent the disease, there will always be people who are simply not susceptible to it. So this concept of susceptibility is vital to our understanding of illness and health, and, to the homeopath, important to the understanding of the onset of disease and the selection of the most appropriate treatment.

After attempting to understand the onset of the problem and the cause, if possible, the homeopath then considers the patient's symptoms of illness. In the case of my student, he takes the idea of the backache and attempts to understand it as best he can. Where exactly in the back does it hurt? What is the sensation of the pain? What makes the pain feel better or worse? What is the patient's mood and behavior when in pain? And what other changes have occurred during this period of time in which the patient has had the backache?

By finding out all this information and by observing the patient, how he moves, how he uses his body while in pain, and then by examining the patient, the homeopath can give a remedy that best deals with the exact nature of this particular patient and his particular backache and not just with the overall concept of "backache" itself. This is a primary difference between homeopathic and allopathic medicine. Homeopathic medicine may use any one of dozens of remedies for the treatment of the backache. Allopathic medicine sticks with the painkillers and the anti-inflammatories. Because the homeopathic remedy targets both the specific symptoms of the back pain and that pain within the context of the patient as a whole being (especially in cases of chronic pain), the treatment is specifically geared to the patient. It is the patient who is being treated, not just his backache. This is what makes homeopathic treatments both safer—in that they are specific to the needs of the individual patient—and more effective—in that they are completely individualized to the needs of this one specific patient.

That's why I end up shaking my head and saying, "That's not how it works," so often: because moving from allopathy to homeopathy involves a *fundamental* shift in thinking. One that involves letting go of the idea of medicine as quid pro quo. One that stops using the physician as a pill dispenser, who you approach, hands, out, saying only, "I have a backache," and then wait expectantly for the pills that will surely follow.

CHAPTER 4

The First Principle of Homeopathic Healing: Similarity

In previous chapters I have already stated this principle as "like cures like"—that the medicine whose actions are closest to the totality of a patient's symptoms of illness will be the medicine of best choice in restoring that patient to health. It is because of the principle of Similarity that homeopathic remedies work in accordance with the body's own healing mechanism. Let's stop and think for a moment about why this is the case.

Actually, you already know everything you need to about how healing takes place, about our own inborn ability to heal. It's a principle of physics you learned in junior high science class: Isaac Newton's Third Law of Motion. Stated simply, this universal principle is "for every action, there is an equal and opposite reaction." This principle is not only true on a universal scale, it is true on the individual human scale as well.

And it points to another fundamental difference between homeopathic and allopathic medicine.

Equal/Opposite

Allopathic medicine, for our purposes here, can be said to be an *active* form of medicine. What I mean by this is that allopathic medicines are chosen and used because of their more or less predictable primary action. To put it into Newton's terms, an allopathic medicine is chosen because it has a powerful impact upon the human body. For the patient whose nose is running because of a cold, a medicine is chosen whose impact is to dry up the sinuses. For the patient who cannot sleep, a medicine is given whose impact is to cause drowsiness. For the patient in pain, a medicine is given that inhibits the patient's ability to experience pain. Always, the medicine is given to counter the symptoms at hand. And always, the medicine is chosen for the sake of its primary action, the initial impact of the medicine.

But what does the body do as a result of that impact? Remember Newton's Third Law—it pushes back. Any motion in one direction is met with an equal and opposite reaction, a shove in the opposite direction. And so you will see it illustrated again and again. Allopathic sleep aides work well the first night and the second. Over time, as the body begins to react against their actions, more and more of the drug will be needed to create the same effect. This is true whether the medicine is a painkiller, a sleep aid, an antibiotic, or any other form of allopathic medicine. The body's natural response to anything that creates a change is to push back against the change, and, in doing so, the body's reaction to allopathic treatment is to move further and further in the direction of the illness and not of health.

Homeopathy works in the opposite manner and, for our purposes here may be said to be a *reactive* form of medicine. This is because the homeopath sees symptoms as the body's reaction to stress, to some susceptibility in the first place. He then works with the symptoms and not against them. The patient who cannot sleep is given a remedy whose actions include causing sleeplessness—the remedy Coffea, made from coffee, is one obvious example. The patient in pain is given a remedy that has been proven to cause not just pain in general, but the exact same sensation of pain in the same area of the body in healthy people. The remedy Rhus Toxicodendron, made from poison ivy, is an example, as it is commonly used for pains like backache when the patient feels the greatest pain on first motion and the pain is lessened by slow, steady movement of the afflicted part of the body. Another remedy, Hypericum, might be used in the case of a patient with pain that runs along a nerve, as in cases involving sciatica.

But it is always the same: *like cures like.* Why? Because when a homeopath gives a remedy that is as similar as can be to the patient's own symptoms of illness, the action of the remedy triggers an equal and opposite response, just as it did with the allopathic treatment. Only, because the homeopathic remedy works in accordance with the symptoms of sleeplessness, pain or sore throat, cold, fever, and so on, the immune system's equal response in the opposite direction actually triggers a healing response. The symptoms are shoved out of the body and, as a result, the sleepless patient sleeps, the achy patient is soothed (the pain is removed, not numbed) and that patient with a cold or flu swiftly recovers. Nothing is suppressed, nothing is numbed, denied, or shoved down. Everything is brought back into balance. Homeopathic remedies work by strengthening the body's own immune response, which is itself a reactive principle. When the immune system identifies a threat, it takes action, and in taking action, it creates fevers, mucus flow, pain, sleeplessness, or other symptom—all as a means of bringing the body back into balance. All as a means of healing. When the body lacks the vital strength to complete the healing response, homeopathic remedies give the body's own natural immunity a boost, allowing the patient's own system to heal itself. Once the healing has taken place, there is no further need for treatment.

Good News/Bad News

Homeopathic treatment can be said to involve a little bad news along with the good news. The good news is that the patient who is treated homeopathically will recover swiftly and will experience a boost to his or her general vitality that will help keep them healthier in general in the future. The bad news is that, when a patient is treated homeopathically, they do not get to pretend that they are not sick. While the patient with a cold will recover much more swiftly and the cold symptoms themselves will be lighter and more easily tolerated, the symptoms will not be numbed—there will be no suppression of the symptoms at all. The patient will have to experience his or her cold before the point of recovery. This can be confusing to those who were raised in a culture in which only the poor are forced to actually have the disease that they are having. In which the rich are always able to find a pill that will inhibit their experience of their discomfort.

Homeopaths know what therapists also know, however—that no one ever got healthy by living in denial. Just as the patient who hates his parent and who refuses to acknowledge his feelings or deal with them will not be strengthened as a person by denying of his emotions, the patient whose medication suppresses his symptoms instead of actually treating them will find, in time, that he has been weakened by his treatments, not strengthened. Those symptoms that have been suppressed deeper into the system will have to reoccur, in some manner, at some time. The allopathic treatments that shove down a patient's discomfort will only create a greater form of discomfort later on.

The best news about the good-news-bad-news of homeopathy is that when a patient has been appropriately treated and the symptoms cleared, they have been cleared away for good. Nothing has been suppressed and the future points to greater health, not more disease.

Like Cures Like—Getting It Right

In today's world, we are finding that even this—the core principle by which homeopathic remedies work and the method by which remedies are appropriately selected—is being bastardized. More and more, the shelves of our health food stores are stocked with remedies that claim to be homeopathic and yet are bottled for the treatment of colds, influenza, stomach upset, headaches, teething pains, acne, and so forth. Think for a moment: can any "homeopathic" medicine that is being suggested as a medicine for a specific condition ever truly be homeopathic? When we say "like cures like" aren't we carrying along with that the fact that we never, in homeopathic treatments, treat a disease, but always treat a patient who happens to have a set number of unique symptoms?

Some companies have learned that if they dumb down the process by which a homeopathic remedy is selected and make it more or less paint by numbers by packaging a remedy (or mixed remedies—see the next chapter for this) as being for the treatment of a specific illness they will sell more products. That may well be true, but it is incorrect in terms of homoeopathic philosophy and in terms of moral behavior.

While I'm on the subject of labeling, if you look on any container of any single homeopathic remedy you will find a list of the things that the remedy typically treats. Why is that?

The reason is that we live in an allopathic world. And the government agencies, in this case the Food and Drug Administration, tend to fall in lockstep with the allopathic culture as well. Therefore, it is required by law, because homeopathic remedies are considered legal over-the-counter medications in the United States, that each bottle or tube of remedies list indications for their use. It may fly in the face of the practice of homeopathic medicine, but each tube of Sulphur must list that it is a nice remedy for those who are suffering from "skin rash worsened by heat and water." True enough, as far as it goes, but hardly worth the ink that it takes to print it.

In the same way, each tube or bottle of homeopathic medication must have an expiration date printed on it. This again is because homeopathic medicines, when placed on the counters of drug stores or health food stores, must play by the allopath's rules. Well stored— which is to say that if the remedies are stored in a moderate climate, well away from direct sunlight or electromagnetic pulses (it is never a good idea to store them in a bowl on top of the microwave, for instance)—homeopathic remedies will not lose their potency for years beyond their printed expiration date. Have no fear; the remedy you buy today will be potent for years to come.

CHAPTER 5

The Second Principle of Homoeopathic Healing: Simplicity

The principle of Simplicity when it comes to medicine is the easiest concept to explain but the hardest to adhere to, especially in our culture. We have been trained since birth to think that more is always better, especially when it comes to medicine. But the principle of Simplicity states that, in homeopathic treatments, we should always use just one medicine at a time.

In fact, Samuel Hahnemann so believed in this principle of Simplicity that he thought that much of the toxicity of allopathic medicine could be removed if allopaths could be convinced to follow it as well. Allopathic medicines, used singly, would be safer and more effective.

However, in the ongoing friction between allopathic and homeopathic practitioners, more homeopaths have been convinced to give up this principle than allopaths have been convinced to follow it. Part of this is cultural, of course, and reflects the Western notion that more of anything is better than less. And part of it may well reflect on just how hard the homeopath's job can be—searching for and finding the best single remedy for a given patient is not an easy task. Whatever the reason, the fact remains that, in the world today, the principle of Simplicity is the one that is most commonly broken in the name of "modern" medicine.

Practitioners will say that the world today is more complex than it was in Hahnemann's day. That our environment is more polluted. That our diseases have been suppressed by generations of allopathic treatments. That patients are harder to cure today than they were two hundred years ago.

And all of this is true. I don't argue with any of it. But none of these reasons are good enough, sufficient enough, for skilled homeopathic practitioners to abandon the core principles of the art. In fact, the complexity of our modern world should make our homeopaths all the more likely to cling to the simplicity of homeopathic treatment, not abandon it.

The principle of Simplicity is fixed. It is a core tenet of homeopathic practice. And the moment the rule is relaxed or ignored and remedies are given in combination, the treatment, however effective or ineffective it may be, ceases to be truly homeopathic.

One Remedy at a Time

Why is this principle so important—why do homeopaths give only one remedy at a time?

The answer to this again goes back to the fact that every medicine has more than one action. It does more than one thing. And to the fact that each patient is an individual and each patient's system is unique, both in illness and in health.

Therefore, it is important that the medical practitioner be as watchful as can be. Since the job of any medicine is to create changes, it is largely the job of the practitioner to choose the medicine that will create the best possible changes. And since every medicine creates myriad changes, both "good" and "bad" (good and bad both being relative terms that shift from patient to patient, illness to illness), only by giving one medicine at a time can the practitioner keep track of the changes. Only by giving one medicine at a time can any physician know whether or not his patient is getting better.

Think about what happens, in either allopathic or homeopathic treatments, when you layer one medicine upon another. If the first medicine does twelve different things—has a dozen forms of impact upon the body, mind, and emotions—and the second medicine does ten things, how well can any practitioner tell which medicine has done what? And as you add more and more medicines, so much more chaos will result.

Polypharmacy

Indeed, when medicines are layered on top of each other—a process known as polypharmacy, which Hahnemann denounces equally in all forms of medicine—it not only becomes impossible to know which medicines are helping and which medicines are harming the patient, but it also becomes impossible to tell if two or more medicines are creating new artificial diseases along side of the naturally occurring symptoms. This is, in fact, so common an occurrence in allopathic medicine that allopaths have given it a name. *Iatrogenic* diseases are those that are caused, not by viruses or bacteria, but by medicines that have been given in the treatment of disease. The very fact that the term exists, or needs to exist, should be cause for outrage on the part of patients. And the fact that allopaths accept the existence of iatrogenic diseases, just as they consider side effects to be part of normal and sensible medical treatments should, in my opinion, send millions of patients of allopathic doctors running for the door.

Homeopaths give one remedy at a time so that the effects of that remedy can be studied and traced, and so that the administration of the next dose of medicine can be administered appropriately. Only by giving a single dose of a single remedy can the physician be sure to know when to give the next dose, and in what potency (for notes on potency and dosage, turn to the next chapter). Whenever we begin to practice a form of half-homeopathy in which homeopathic remedies are mixed and layered as allopathic drugs tend to be, we create a situation in which the case becomes increasingly muddled, until it can reach the point at which the practitioner cannot know what to do next. At worst, the patient who has been treated with multiple remedies for long enough can have his case so muddled that homeopathic treatment may no longer be an option.

Combination Remedies

The shelves of our health food stores are loaded with boxes of supposedly homeopathic medicines in which several remedies are combined on one tablet. These are known as combination or mixed remedies. And while I do not speak to their efficacy—in the short term, they work well enough and are not terribly dangerous—I do want you to be aware that they are not and cannot be called homeopathic. Homeopathic treatments always involve the use of one remedy at a time. When the first remedy has done all it can—when the patient's symptoms have shifted so that they are no longer similar to those that the remedy creates—then, if the patient has not been made well, another remedy must be selected, again on the basis of similarity.

When a combination remedy is given, especially in cases involving chronic conditions, all the remedies in the combination have some effect on the patient's system. All cause changes over time. And think about it for a moment—think about the potential for harm if a mixture of remedies is taken over a period of time. Think about how chaotic the patient's symptoms can potentially become and hard it can be to tell which remedy has caused what change.

I am not overly concerned when a patient with a cold takes a combination remedy for colds and coughs for a day or two, but when supposedly homeopathic practitioners begin to give combinations of many different remedies for the treatment of chronic conditions like allergies, I become deeply concerned. I cannot predict what these treatments might do. I cannot say whether they will be totally safe or effective or not. I can only say, clearly and distinctly, that they are not homeopathic.

CHAPTER 6

The Third Principle of Homeopathic Healing: Minimum

It is always the goal of homeopathic treatment that the patient be healed, nothing less. It is not the goal of homeopathic treatment that the disease be managed or that the patient take a remedy or group of remedies each day for the rest of his life. Those are allopathic concepts. The allopath believes that that which cannot be cured—to use the allopath's word—must be managed. And if medicines cannot be found to cure a disease, then medicines must be found to manage it, to keep it just under control enough that the patient survives to swallow some more pills tomorrow, no matter how restricted or unhappy the patient's life and no matter how toxic and ineffective his medicine.

Homeopaths think differently.

The principle of Minimum states two things, each of which is a promise that, once homeopathic treatment has begun, the goal of that treatment is the rapid, gentle, and permanent restoration of health, followed by the end of treatment. Homeopathic treatments are meant to be finite, because they are meant to actually be curative, to put it in allopathic terms once more.

Dosage

Just as homeopathic treatments always begin with a single remedy, they also begin with a single dose. Because the patient is an individual and because the homeopath is treating that individual patient and not his or her disease, the practitioner always undertakes the treatment with just one dose of the selected remedy. The practitioner then waits a period of time—determined both by the severity of the situation at hand and by the remedy of choice (some remedies work faster than others, and some must be repeated more often than others, while some work best in single dose)—before determining the next dose.

If the first dose of the selected remedy clears away the patient's symptoms, no second dose should be given. This can be hard to grasp for those of us who were raised in an allopathic culture. I have never known an allopath who found a single dose of *anything* to be suffi-cient, but the homeopath is guided by the patient and by his or her symptoms.

First and foremost, the practitioner is looking for a change in the symptoms—*either for better or worse*. Especially in simple acute cases, the symptoms will often grow a little worse before they dramatically improve. This is referred to as an *aggravation*. As the remedy stirs the patient's immunity, the symptoms—which are the sign that the patient's immune system is seeking to right itself—may grow a bit more intense for a brief period of time. This is a sign that the remedy is working.

Sometimes there is no aggravation. Instead, the patient may fall into a quiet gentle sleep. This is another sign of improvement. They will likely awaken feeling much better. But it is the shift in symptoms and in the patient's demeanor that the practitioner is looking for, and not necessarily the total resolution of the case in the first few minutes.

Should the patient's condition show no signs of change whatso-ever, it is likely that the remedy given was not similar enough in its action to work with the symptoms at hand. Or that the right remedy was given in too low a potency. In either case, the practitioner should, while still watching the patient for signs of change, consider another remedy or an adjustment in potency.

After the first shift in symptoms, the practitioner will then look for signs of improvement. A gentle sleep, as has been noted, is one of these, as is simply the lifting of symptoms. Often, the patient himself will not be aware of how improved he may be after a single dose of the remedy. In that the homeopathic remedy has no side effects, causes no numbness or disorientation, the patient may need to have it pointed out to him that he has not sneezed for over an hour or that his voice, once hoarse, now sounds very much like his own normal voice.

If the shift in symptoms is slight, the remedy may be repeated, perhaps with the potency increased. But once improvement has begun, no further doses should be given unless or until the improvement begins to fade and symptoms begin to return. Homeopathic remedies should always be given on an "as needed" basis—no more, no less.

Potency

The idea of potency—how powerful a dose of a particular remedy—is key both to our understanding of the philosophy of homeopathy as well as to its practice. When choosing a potency, the homeopath seeks once more to match the symptoms of the patient and then to give a remedy that is slightly more powerful than the natural disease state. The idea is to artificially boost the threat to the immune system, and, in doing so, to encourage the body's own healing mechanism to work harder, to rise up in equal and opposite action against the remedy's impact. In doing so, the body eliminates the natural symptoms more efficiently, and when the action of the remedy fades, health and balance are restored. It is therefore very important for the practitioner— whether a medical professional dealing with a serious, even life-threatening disease or a lay practitioner treating his or her own child who has an earache or fever—to learn to judge the potency correctly.

Should the practitioner give too high a potency, he may stir up the symptoms more than is needed and create a greater aggravation than necessary. While this is not dangerous, it can be uncomfortable for the patient.

Should the practitioner give too low a potency, the patient's response may be so subtle that the practitioner mistakenly comes to believe that he has given the wrong remedy and moves on to another when he sees no apparent response in the patient's symptoms.

When the potency is right, the response is clear: the patient improves. Again, the meaning of that word can be a bit tricky, because improvement can be as individualized as the experience of the disease symptoms themselves. What I tend to look for is a general improvement rather than an improvement of symptoms. It can take a little time for those to clear away. But the patient will usually receive a boost to his system. Even if you were treating him for a headache and he still has the headache after taking the remedy, he might say that he can handle the pain better, or that, in general, he feels better, even in spite of the pain. Statements like these are a clear sign that improvement has begun, and, remember, once improvement begins, the best thing to do is to withhold the next dose and just wait and give the remedy a chance to work.

More homeopathic cases are spoiled by giving the remedy too often then by giving it too little.

What do I mean by this? I mean that, just as giving a combination of remedies can confuse a case, giving a single remedy—even the right remedy—too often can confuse things as well. It is a process called *proving.*

As I have noted above, the concept of Similarity tells us that we must, as best we can, match the symptoms the patient is experiencing to the total actions of a specific single remedy. The better the match, the more effective the treatment.

But what happens if you give the wrong remedy—one that is not similar in its action to the patient's symptoms? As I indicated earlier, in the vast majority of cases, nothing whatsoever will happen. The remedy will not act at all because it is not is a state of similarity to the patient or his symptoms. But if you continue to give a remedy over and over, even if it is in no way similar to the patient or his symptoms, the remedy will begin to artificially graft the symptoms it creates onto the patient.

Again, this is not dangerous, merely unpleasant. If you stop giving the remedy, the symptoms it creates will fade. But even if you give the right remedy too often, you will first see an improvement in which the symptoms fade, followed by a mysterious reappearance of the symptoms, returning not naturally but artificially, as the result of giving repeated doses of the remedy. This may fool the unskilled practitioner into thinking that they gave the wrong remedy and send them rushing to their homeopathic kits, when all they need to do is to stop giving the remedy and the symptoms will fade and the patient will be made well.

Let me say it again: homeopathic remedies are given as needed. If the remedy works for only a few minutes and then the symptoms return, repeat the dose. If the patient improves and does not need another dose of the remedy, do not give another dose. (Note: in the first case I described above in which the remedy needed to be repeated very often to continue working, this is an indication that a higher potency was needed.)

Homeopathic Remedies in Their Potencies

Homeopathic potencies are based upon the process of dilution.

It is a very simple concept. Samuel Hahnemann, both during the time in which he was studying medicine at the University of Vienna and afterward, when he established a traditional allopathic medical practice in the region of the Hartz Mountains in Germany, noticed again and again that, as he put it, more patients were dying of their medical treatments than were dying from their diseases.

To try and find a way in which he could make the standard allopathic drugs of his day less toxic, Hahnemann began to simply dilute them in water. He did this systematically, at first taking one part of the medicinal substance and mixing it with nine parts water, for a scale of dilutions that would be referred to as the "X" scale—X being the Roman numeral for ten—and then later by taking one part substance and mixing it with ninety-nine parts water in the creation of the "C" scale—C being the Roman numeral for one hundred.

What he found seemed counter-intuitive. The more diluted the substance became, the less toxic it became. That much was no surprise. What was surprising was that the more and more diluted it became, the more and more powerful it became as a healing agent. It was as if in washing away the substance, he was uncovering more and more the life force of the natural substance that could be used to restore patients to health.

Further, Samuel Hahnemann in his clinical trials discovered that remedies that had been shaken in their liquid state worked more powerfully than those that had not. And so in establishing his protocols for what he called the *potentizing* of natural substances into homeopathic remedies, he developed a two-step process, involving both dilution and *succussion,* or shaking. Note that many homeopathic remedies are diluted to the point at which no molecules of the original substance remain. This is what makes substances like arsenic, cyanide, and snake venom into nontoxic remedies. With the toxins removed, only the energy signatures of the original substances remain.

Choosing the Right Potency

A simple rule of thumb for choosing the right potency has to do with what types of symptoms the patient has. By this I mean, the more the patient's symptoms are based in the physical body, the lower the remedy's potency should be. A patient with a rash, for instance, should be given a very low potency, because the aggravation of a rash will tend to spread it all over the body—the patient will still get well, but will be very unhappy with his treatment. So I'd give a very low potency, even perhaps a 6X or a 9X. (Remember, because the X potencies are diluted only into tenths, they are much less potent than the C scale remedies.)

But the more the patient's mood and thought process are being disrupted—the more the symptoms affect the invisible and intangible parts of the body—the higher the needed potency. Most commonly, homeopathic remedies are given in the 30C potency. Is that because it is the "best" potency? No. It is because it is the most commonly available potency.

The 30C potency is a good basic choice for symptoms that primarily affect the physical body, but that also can include a bad mood or a hazy thought process or some other indication that the emotional/ mental self is also affected. For this reason, it is an excellent potency for most common household complaints like simple mechanical injuries, upper respiratory conditions, and simple joint pain. Professional practitioners may use much higher potencies with excellent results, but most home kits sold in health food stores or by homeopathic pharmacies will contain remedies in the 30C potency and lower.

In closing, never underestimate the power of a homeopathic remedy. Even in low potencies and single doses, they can have dramatic results. Just because they come in sweet milk sugar pellets (Hahnemann was the first to place his remedies in liquid form onto milk sugar pellets that he then gave to his patients. He chose milk sugar to carry his remedies' potencies because he found milk sugar to be both pleasant and, as a substance, nearly completely benign and nonmedicinal, making it the ideal container for his remedies.) does not mean that they are candy. All homeopathic home kits need to be treated with respect and safely stored where small hands cannot reach them.

CHAPTER 7

The Goals of Homeopathic Treatment

The most basic goal of any medical treatment is to help patients feel better. They come into the doctor's office reporting some pain, some set of symptoms, and they want help in feeling better, getting past those symptoms of discomfort.

There are, however, three levels of homeopathic treatment, each with its own goal and each with its own demands in terms of skill in case taking and case management.

Acute Treatments

Acute illnesses are those that, by their very nature, are self-limiting. They appear, flare up for a time, and then fade away. Most of the time, the patient would recover without any sort of medical intervention.

But this is not always the case. While many acute illnesses are colds, sore throats, and earaches, others, like influenza, can be both acute and potentially very dangerous. The great flu outbreak of the early part of the last century is an example of an acute illness that killed millions worldwide.

Most of the time, however, the case taking required in order to find the right remedy for an acute illness is fairly simple. All the practitioner has to do is to uncover how the patient has changed, in terms of symptoms in body, mind, and emotions, since the onset of the illness. Once the number and type of symptoms associated with the illness are gathered and considered, the practitioner can decide upon the remedy. Chief among the symptoms considered are:

- Onset: The circumstances during which the illness began, including weather conditions, time of day or night, the patient's level of stress, and so on.

- Sensation: The character of symptom or pain—here the symptom is subjective in nature: whether the specific pain is dull or throbbing, for example.

- Location: The specific location of pain; a headache in the forehead, for example, as opposed to a headache in the temples.

- Duration: How long a symptom has occurred and the order of appearance of each symptom. This is helpful in determining how the healing will take place, as usually the first symptom to arrive is the last to go.

- Modalities: The specific conditions by which each symptom is made better or worse: temperature, weather conditions, time of day or night, body positions, and so on.

- General Modalities: Just as it is helpful to know what makes each symptom feel better or worse, if is very helpful to know what makes the patient as a whole feel better or worse. The patient who feels better when alone will need a different remedy from the patient who needs constant company, just as the need to be covered up tight suggests a different remedy from the need to kick off the covers at night.

By gathering this information, the homeopathic practitioner can most often very quickly identify the required remedy. The goal of the acute treatment is a simple one, and is the most similar to that of allopathic medicine as you will find in homeopathic treatments: to restore the patient to the level of health that he enjoyed before the onset of the illness. Therefore, if the patient had panic attacks and asthma before the treatment, he will still have them after the treatment. Acute treatments center on the changes that have taken place in the patient's life only recently and the remedies selected are selected on the basis of those changes (symptoms) only.

To be effective in acute treatments, the practitioner must have the ability to see the remedies embodied in human flesh. He must have an understanding of the remedies that allows him to make quick decisions largely based upon objective symptoms that can be seen or measured, such as skin that is brightly colored or pale, a tongue that is swollen, or mucus that is watery as opposed to thick and colored. While the ailments that fall under the category of acute homeopathy are usually benign enough to be treated by the student of homeopathy, it is important to understand that the skilled acute practitioner, like the skilled allopathic emergency room doctor, must have at the ready a great knowledge of acute medicine and his pharmaceutical tools. While this is a different skill set than that needed for the chronic case, it is no less important.

Constitutional Treatments

Constitutional treatments concern themselves with ailments that are more established in the patient's system, with chronic complaints and with strong patterns of negative behavior in the patient's life. Therefore, the practitioner must go deeper in his case taking and must assess the case more carefully when researching the remedy or remedies needed to treat the patient and restore him to health.

While the case taking will involve all the information listed above for acute care, it will also require a detailed look into the life of the patient and his medical history. It will be important to know the onset of any or all symptoms related to the chronic complaint as well as the nature of the patient's general health since childhood and the number and types of other complaints he has experienced.

The goal of constitutional treatment is deeper and wider-ranging than that of acute treatments. The constitutional treatment, in clearing away the long-term symptoms associated with chronic illness, will also clear away layers of suppression and denial that have been put in place by a lifetime of allopathic care. Further, in removing the layers of illness, the patient will not only experience an improvement in the symptoms that led him into treatment, but will find himself strengthened in terms of his immunity, making him far less susceptible to future illness.

It is the domain of the homeopathic medical professional to undertake constitutional treatments, because of the complexity of the treatment and the knowledge both of the healing process and the homeopathic pharmacy required. The student of homeopathy, no matter how skilled, should not undertake such treatments.

Miasmic Treatments

The word miasm itself means *taint*. To Hahnemann, miasms were barriers to successful treatments, walls around aspects of his patients' lives that would not allow his treatments to be wholly successful. Today, we would define a miasm as a genetic predisposition to an illness or set of illnesses. When you see a serious and/or chronic illness affecting several members of the same family, you are typically looking at the effects of a miasm.

Miasms are caused chiefly by suppressive medical treatments. The stronger the allopathic treatment, the deeper the suppression. With the advent of powerful antibiotics and steroids, we have seen an increase in the number of patients needing miasmic care.

This is the deepest level of homeopathic treatment. It requires a very skilled practitioner, one who understands not only the constitutional implications of a patient's symptoms, but the miasmic implications as well. Miasmic treatments can be slow in resolving, but, as with all homeopathic treatments, once the patient has completed treatment, he is completely well. There is no level of suppression of symptoms in homeopathic treatment.

Ironically, when you look at the three levels of homeopathic treatment, you will often find that the acute treatment takes the most remedies and doses of remedies to resolve. A cold, for instance, may require three different remedies, one for each stage of the cold (from onset to mucus flow, from clear mucus flow to when it becomes colored, and, finally, the stage at which the mucus is thick and colored). A constitutional treatment may consist of only one or two remedies, each of which may be given in several different potencies in order to clear away symptoms. A miasmic treatment may consist of a single dose of a single remedy, well selected, that will clear away all miasmic blocks to treatment if allowed to act for a period of time. Once we have the miasmic blockage cleared the treatment would be the same as it would for any other constitutional case.

By understanding the needs of the individual patient and the situation at hand, the homeopathic practitioner can tailor the treatment to balance the patient's life energy, strengthen his immunity, and free him of all his symptoms of illness. All homeopathic treatments require an understanding both of the practice and philosophy of homeopathy as well as knowledge of the thousands of remedies that are a part of the homeopathic pharmacy.

With this knowledge, the sick can be made well. And illnesses large and small—from pebbles to boulders—can be removed. This is the promise that Samuel Hahnemann made in his book, *The Organon of the Healing Art:* that homeopathic treatments will restore the sick to health, in a manner that is rapid, gentle, and permanent. Rapid. Gentle. And permanent.

Lighting the Spark: The Ultimate Goal of Treatment

I've mentioned this before in other books, but it merits repeating. It pertains to all levels of homeopathic treatment. Indeed, it pertains to all medical treatments of all sorts.

Paracelsus, a healer who bridged the gap between alchemist and chemist, said something that stayed with me, as it provides an understanding of the purpose of medicine and the way healing takes place. He said that, when he worked with a patient, he approached the healing process like the process of building a fire in his fireplace. When building a fire, he did not sit and consider the exact amount of fire it would take for the wood to light. No, he said, he just struck a match and allowed the natural process of combustion to take place.

In the same way, when it came to healing, he felt that it was the role of the physician to strike a spark and then allow it to ignite. Because healing, like combustion, is a natural process.

In working with the process, one only has to light a spark, giving the patient a chance to heal himself. And then step back and watch the results, stepping in only as one does when working with a fire—to stir the embers until the process is done.

CHAPTER 8

Popular Misconceptions about Homeopathic Treatment

You hear all sorts of things about homeopathy, about the remedies and their uses and about the way that homeopathic healing takes place. Some of the things you hear are right, others are just plain wrong, still others are just strange and confusing. I thought I'd set the record straight about a few of them:

Homeopathy and Herbal Medicine

I feel that this merits saying one more time—homeopathic medicine is *not* the same thing as herbal medicine. While our modern homeopathic remedies come from the herbal tradition, just as allopathic drugs do, they are not the same thing. In order for a substance—animal, vegetable or mineral—to become a homeopathic remedy, it must go through a two-step process known as potentization, in which the substance is first diluted and then shaken while in its liquid, diluted state. So while some herbal medicines may well be as toxic as any allopathic drug (think of such herbals as belladonna, for example), all homeopathic remedies are rendered safe by the potentization process. Further, while there may be some variation in potency from herbal tincture to herbal tincture, all homeopathic remedies of the same level of potentization, whether 9X, 30C or 1M, are completely identical in terms of action and potency. It is also worth noting that the mindset in using herbal medicines and homeopathic remedies is very different. Herbal medicines are used in the treatment of diseases, and in this way are more like allopathic drugs than homeopathic remedies. Homeopathic remedies are used in the treatment of patients, not diseases, and remedies are selected by matching the totality of a patient's symptoms with the total action of a given remedy. The more similar the remedy is in its action to the symptoms that the patient is experiencing, the more powerfully the remedy will act as a tool for healing.

Antidoting Remedies

A lot of students of homeopathy, especially beginning students of homeopathy, are obsessed with the idea of antidoting a homeopathic treatment. (And by the term "antidoting," I refer to two things, both the halting of treatment that has been begun—eating mint, in some cases, may cause a once-active remedy to stop working at the point at which the mint was eaten—or, in more severe cases, the undoing of treatment and the re-establishment of past symptoms because of a particularly strong reaction to something touched, tasted or smelled.) Many worry that any number of things will antidote them, like mint in a toothpaste or garlic in the spaghetti sauce. Honestly, in my experience, it is not easy to antidote the actions of a remedy. Coffee is most often listed as the chief antidote. But here's the thing. If you drink coffee every day, if it is something that your system is used to, it will not antidote you. It will antidote or at least blunt the action of a remedy only if, like me, you very seldom drink coffee and therefore tend to react strongly to it, if it is sort of medicinal to your system. Hahnemann's concern was that those under homeopathic treatment avoid as many things as possible that have a medicinal effect—that create strong changes in the system. Anything that does can potentially be an issue. You should avoid strong smells, especially if you are allergic to a lot of things. Cheap, chemically produced perfumes can be problematic. Camphor in all its forms is the most guaranteed antidote. Hahnemann used it when a patient got a strong aggravation. You can use it, too. Keep a container of Tiger Balm in the house and, should you give too high a potency, you can have the patient rub the balm on his wrists and breathe in the scent. That will do the trick. But don't use it during a homeopathic treatment that you don't want to antidote.

Storing Remedies

People get overly worried about this as well, some even to the point of not wanting the vials of different remedies to touch, as they believe that they will contaminate each other. But the remedies are simple to store. Just keep them in a temperate place and out of direct sun. Store them with their lids on tight. Do NOT store them on top of a microwave or a refrigerator or any other device that has a strong electro magnetic field. This can ruin the remedies, like direct sunlight can. And while it is fine to store many different remedies together in a box, I never take the last few pellets from one tube and pour them into the next. I'm not sure why—I just don't. I think that, should something have contaminated one, I don't want to contaminate both. We all have our funny ways.

Taking Remedies

There is a good bit of confusion around how many pellets should be taken at a time. The rule of thumb here is that you want to, first of all, be working with a clean tongue—and by this I mean one that has no tastes on it, not one that has just been brushed. You should take a remedy ideally either a good fifteen minutes before eating or drinking (water is the sole exception and may be drunk before, after, or while dosing with remedies) or an hour afterward. Then you just want to use enough pellets to coat the tongue. Usually three to five pellets will do. Some remedies, most notably the homeopathic flu remedy sold by Boiron called Oscillococcinum, are sold in small tubes with very small pellets. These are called "unit doses" and the idea here is that you will take the entire tube of pellets as a single dose. And you certainly may, without harm. But, again, the idea in taking a remedy in pellet form is that you coat the tongue—so with the unit dose, you may, just as you do with other remedies presented on larger pellets, take only the amount of pellets needed to give the tongue a good coating—with the unit doses this usually means about a dozen pellets. This way you will need to buy your remedies infrequently and will still enjoy the full benefits of using them.

The Use of "Aqua Remedies"

Any homeopathic remedy that is sold in pellet form may be dissolved in water to create an "aqua remedy." And these dissolved pellets will do the same work in liquid form that they did in solid. Simply take five or so pellets and dissolve in room-temperature filtered water, about half a glass full. These dissolved remedies have several uses. First, they may be used topically. You may, for instance, dissolve Sulphur and dab the Aqua Sulphur over a rash that is being treated by the remedy, while, at the same time, taking the remedy internally in pellet form. The topical use of the remedy will help speed healing. Or the aqua remedy may be taken internally, in place of the pellets. There are two reasons you might choose to do this. First, if you are quickly running out of pellets and have no convenient way to buy more—say it is the middle of the night and you have a child with an earache—you may dissolve the remedy as instructed above and then stretch out the doses by giving the aqua remedy in place of the pellets. That way, one dose of pellets can be stretched until you can buy more. To use the aqua remedy, get a clean spoon, stir the remedy briskly for a moment and then place a couple of spoonfuls of the remedy on the patient's tongue. Be careful not to touch the remedy on the tongue and then place back in the glass. Have the patient hold the aqua remedy in his or her mouth for a few moments before swallowing. The second reason for dissolving the pellets is to give a slight variance to the potency of the remedy between doses. To do this, don't just stir for a moment, but really give the aqua remedy a very good agitation with the spoon. The more you stir it, the more potent you make the remedy. This will not shift the potency greatly, only very little, but the fact that you are not repeating the exact same remedy time and again will help to make it work a little more effectively. Aqua remedies may be stored in the refrigerator for about a day before they begin to lose their potency. Make sure to keep them tightly covered with a bit of plastic wrap on top of the glass.

Handling Remedies

Again, there is a lot of fear around this. Likely, you have heard that in giving a remedy, you should not touch it yourself, but should just spill a couple pellets into the cap and then tip them onto the patient's tongue. That is correct. But the misconception is that, in touching the remedy, you might spoil it. That's not the problem. The problem is that, in touching the remedy, you dose yourself with it. Your skin, like your tongue, is part of your body. You do not want the remedy to come into contact with your body unless your intent is to dose yourself.

How Homeopathic Healing Takes Place

There are a lot of misconceptions about the homeopathic healing process and, as a result, some treatments that are progressing quite well can be undercut because an expected pattern of healing did not take place. A great homeopath named Constantine Hering once set forth a "law" that stated that homeopathic healing takes place three ways—from the top of the head down to the bottom of the feet, from the inside (the tissues deepest in the body) outward to the skin, and from the most recent symptoms back to the most ancient symptoms. In setting forth Hering's Law, I believe that he was offering a general pattern that he had witnessed clinically, and not trying to set forth a hard-and-fast rule. Healings take place in all sorts of ways. But I've known new students to get very upset if the patient's feet start feeling better first. I say just roll with it. Stay within the principles of homeo-pathic treatment. If improvement begins, then watch and wait before doing anything, giving the next dose of the same remedy, or changing remedies. We all heal in our own way, in our own time. It is the heal-ing that is important, not that it follows a particular pattern.

Real Signs of Improvement

There are misconceptions on this subject, the greatest being that there is one sure sign that can be classified as improvement. As we shall see in the answer to the next question, sometimes symptoms must grow temporarily worse before they can get better. Other times, patients simply fall into a calm, deep sleep, from which they awaken feeling much better. Still other times, patients feel an increase in their energy, while still having the same symptoms. They feel better as a whole being, but still have their headache or sore throat. All of these are good signs. Keep this in mind—what we are looking for when giving a remedy is a change. Any change at first. As I said, patients may find their symptoms getting a bit worse on taking the remedy, or may feel better, or may relax into sleep when they have been unable to rest before. In all these cases, within minutes of taking the remedy—sometimes while it is still dissolving on the tongue—the patient will feel some sort of change as a result of taking the remedy. This is the first sign that it is working. From here, the practitioner must watch and wait in order to know when or if to give the remedy again. Remember, while any sort of change is a sign that you have given a remedy whose action is similar enough to have impact, ultimately, we are looking for an improvement of the actual symptoms. In cases of acute illness, this improvement should begin within minutes or, at the longest, hours of giving the remedy. And especially in acute cases, the remedy may have to be repeated to bring about an improvement. But once improvement has begun, it is important to remember to stop giving the remedy. Only if the improvement begins to fade, if the symptoms begin to grow stronger again, should you repeat the remedy once improvement has begun. More homeopathic cases are spoiled by giving the remedy too often or by giving too many different remedies than by giving the remedy less often than needed. If you must err, err on the side of giving too little and not too much.

The Inevitability of Aggravations

This is another hotly debated topic. In my experience, it depends upon the nature of the illness and the strength of the patient's vitality. Aggravations—which are the temporary worsening of the symptoms the patient already has before they begin to dramatically improve—are most likely in acute cases. Therefore, the patient who is suffering from a cold will be very likely to sneeze or to have his sore throat get a little worse before it gets a whole lot better. And the patient who is basically well and strong, but who is wrestling with a temporary and self-limiting ailment, is more likely to have an aggravation because his vitality is basically intact and very strong. It pushes back against the remedy (the "equal and opposite reaction" that is inevitable) in such a way that the symptoms flare due to the immune response and then, as the remedy completes its work, drop off dramatically. On the other hand, the patient who is frail, in whom the life force is very weak, will be less likely to have dramatic aggravations. However, when the vitality is known to be weak, great care must be taken in undertaking any form of treatment, whether homeopathic or allopathic. Only those who are highly skilled at any medical art should be treating them. In cases of chronic conditions of all sorts, from migraines to chronic pain to allergies, the aggravation does not typically come at the beginning of treatment, but, instead, at the end. While the patient may be greatly improved for several months, there will usually be a time during which the old symptoms flare suddenly and without warning. The unskilled practitioner will panic and give higher doses of the same remedy or, worse, a new remedy, thinking that the treatment has failed. The skilled practitioner will see the sudden temporary flare-up as a sign that the need for treatment is about over and the patient's improvement will soon be permanent. This aggravation is a sign that the patient's being is at last throwing off the pattern of chronic symptoms and moving forward into a new and healthier pattern of being. If this aggravation is left untreated, it will soon fade and the improvement will return.

Homeopathy Is Too Complicated for Me to Learn

This is perhaps the greatest misconception of all. True, the homeopath seeks to make every treatment one that is fully individualized to the needs of the patient and always treats the patient and never the disease. And, it is true that the homeopath must therefore consider many different remedies as possibilities and needs to have a strong understanding of material medica. And, it is also true that the homeopath, whether lay homeopath or professional, must learn case management and must oversee and conclude cases with wisdom and compassion. But what is not true is that this is beyond your abilities. The basic rule of thumb is to never attempt to treat any condition that you do not understand—that you always have a basic grasp of the nature of the illness and that you have sufficient understanding of the symptoms at hand. If this means that you are only skilled enough to treat patients with runny noses and sore throats, then that is what you should be doing, nothing more. A good homeopath—again, layperson or professional—knows his or her limits and stays within them. There is plenty of time to study later, when all is well. During a medical crisis, no matter how small, all attention must be given to the patient and all must work for his or her restoration of health in the way that is most rapid, gentle and permanent. If that means calling a doctor, then, by all means, make that call. But if you can learn just a little about the philosophy and practice of homeopathy, think of all the good you can do. As one of my teachers once reminded me years ago—at a time when I was discouraged, thinking that I could never learn all the things a homeopath needs to know—when she looked me in the eye and asked if I had a loved one who had a cold, would I know what to do? "Yes," I said, a little insulted in her selection of an ailment, as I considered colds to be an easy thing to treat. "Well, then," she said to me, "Think of how that sets you apart from all the doctors whose medicines do nothing at all when treating a cold, except to cover up the symptoms for a while. You know how to actually help someone get better when they have a cold! How many allopaths can say the same thing?"

Think about it. Think about all the good you can do with just a little foundation in homeopathic philosophy and a solid knowledge of just a few homeopathic remedies. You may be treating only earaches and skinned knees, but think of the suffering you are soothing and of the great gift of health you are giving.

Education knows no boundary. There is no limit to what you can learn, to your ability to understand the nature of healing and how it takes place. And each bit of learning allows you to give a bit more, and a bit more, and a bit more. To have the ability to help people heal—what gift can be greater than that?

And it is something you can learn, knowledge you can have—if you just reach for it, and grasp it. This book is just a primer, just the smallest of first steps. If you find that you are interested in learning more, just turn the page. What follows is a small directory of resources that can help you with your study of homeopathy or your search for the best homeopathic practitioner for your needs. Either way, a global homeopathic community awaits. You only have to make yourself known.

A Concise Resource Guide to Homeopathy

Books About Homeopathy

This is only a brief list of books available on subjects related to home-opathy, so I have tried to select those that I have found, over the years, to have been of the most value to me.

Lectures on Homeopathic Philosophy, by James Tyler Kent. Reprint edition. Berkley: North Atlantic, 1979. For my money, when it comes to learning about the practice of homeopathy as it is meant to be practiced, it all comes down to the work of two men—Hahnemann and Kent. This book is essential to the understanding of the philosophy of homeopathic medicine and the ramifica-tions of its practice. A must-have book, and one that any serious student of homeopathy will refer to again and again.

The Science of Homeopathy, by George Vithoulkas. New York: Grove, 1980. This was a groundbreaking work when it was first published, in that it considered homeopathy from the scientific point of view. In that modern science has bro-ken the boundaries of what had, heretofore, the invisible aspects of nature, Vithoulkas makes a powerful statement of just how and why homeopathy works by considering homeopathy through the prism of (then) modern physics. Now, over a quarter century later, the book has taken on a retro aspect, but is still worth reading.

Psyche and Substance: Essays on Homeopathy in the Light of Jungian Psychology, by Edward C. Whitmont. Berkeley: North Atlantic, 1991. If I were to say flat out that this is one of the best books ever written on the subject of homeopathy, I might be revealing my own personal bias, but I would also be stating simple fact. No other homeopath of my acquaintance ever impressed me as Whitmont did. His viewpoint is unique and his writing is excellent.

The Alchemy of Healing: Psyche and Soma, by Edward C. Whitmont. Berkley: North Atlantic, 1993. If possible, this is even a better book than Whitmont's first. It is as good, at least. Whitmont was one of the best writers ever to deal with topics related to homeopathy. And this book is Whitmont writing at the top of his game.

Divided Legacy: A History of the Schism in Medical Thought, by Harris Coulter. 4 volumes. Berkeley: North Atlantic, 1975, 1977, 1981, 1994. Let's face it, these four volumes are not an easy read. What you get as your reward if you make it through, however, will enlighten you. Coulter gives his readers the complete history of homeopathy in the United States: how and why homeopathy went from a thriving medical practice to a fringe alternative medicine.

The Patient, Not the Cure: The Challenge of Homeopathy, by Margery Blackie. Santa Barbara: Woodbridge Press, 1978. Blackie's viewpoint can best be summed up by her brief statement: "Homeopathy is not a philosophy, it is a principle." Her book reminds us that homeopathic medicine is based upon an immutable foundation and that its practice, therefore, should always adhere to the laws of cure. The title reminds us of just what it is that makes homeopathic medicine so difficult to practice—the fact that we are always and forever treating people, and never their diseases. As the book (and an amusing photograph inside the cover) reminds us, Blackie once served as the physician to Britain's Queen Elizabeth II, back when that was something to brag about.

A Dictionary of Homeopathic Medical Terminology, by Jay Yasgur. Greenville, PA: Van Hoy Publishers, 1992. This little book will be of great help to you, as it acts as a bridge between the arcane medical jargon used in many repertories and materia medicas and the English language as it is spoken today. It also supplies brief biographical sketches of those who shaped the practice of homeopathy.

The Healing Enigma: Demystifying Homeopathy, by Vinton McCabe. Laguna Beach, CA: Basic Health Publications, 2006. I put more than a quarter of a century's experience of teaching students the philosophy of homeopathic medicine into this book. Part memoir, part history, *The Healing Enigma* is an in-depth look at how homeopathy works and how it can change your life.

Home Guides

Practical Homeopathy, by Vinton McCabe. New York: St. Martin's, 2000. At first I thought that I should not list any of my own books on this resource list, but I am truly proud of this book. I worked hard to not only give a working materia medica for the fifty remedies most commonly used in household emergencies, but also to flesh out the practice of homeopathy as it applies to acute situations. This book is based upon twenty year's worth of my own notes and observations.

Household Homeopathy, by Vinton McCabe. Laguna Beach, CA: Basic Health Publications, 2005. This book is largely based upon the writings of American homeopath John Scudder and is likely the most in-depth book on acute treatments available today. Based on McCabe's teaching notes, it stresses the use of objective symptoms in the selection of homeopathic remedies.

Homeopathic Medicine at Home: Natural Remedies for Everyday Ailments and Minor Injuries by Maesimund B. Panos and Jane Heimlich. Los Angeles: Tarcher, 1976. This was the first homeopathic home guide that I ever owned and was the book that has launched so many others in the modern age. Panos and Heimlich looked back to a time over a hundred years ago, when many homeopaths published little volumes of suggested remedies for home use. They took this information into a new century and with information relating to the American home and family. This is still one of the best home guides and one of the easiest to use.

The Family Guide to Homeopathy: Symptoms and Natural Solutions, by Andrew Lockie. New York: Simon and Schuster Fireside, 1993. I've always really liked this exhaustive work by a British practitioner. Lockie takes almost a naturopathic approach to home health care in this book, and gives not only the suggested homeopathic remedies to choose from, but also important rules for first aid and other "nonhomeopathic" information.

The Complete Homeopathy Handbook: Safe and Effective Ways to Treat Fevers, Coughs, Colds and Sore Throats, Childhood Ailments, Food Poisoning, Flu, and a Wide Range of Everyday Complaints, by Miranda Castro. New York: St Martin's, 1990. The subtitle says it all. In what is, in my opinion, her best book, Castro gives good insight into the remedies that are most commonly associated with the included maladies. She is particularly good at including important emotional and mental symptoms.

Homeopathy for Pregnancy, Birth and Your Baby's First Year, by Miranda Castro. New York: St. Martin's, 1993. While I am not a woman and have no children, I can still recognize that Miranda Castro writes about the subject as it relates to homeopathy with a warmth and humor all too often missing from these books. This excellent guide lives up to its title, giving exhaustive information on the issues surrounding pregnancy and birth, as well as postnatal care and early childhood healthcare.

For other books related to women's health and childbirth, consider:

The Women's Guide to Homeopathy, by Andrew Lockie and Nicola Geddes. New York: St. Martin's, 1994.

Natural Healing for Women, by Susan Curtis and Romy Fraser. London: Pandora, 1991.

Homeopathic Medicine for Pregnancy and Childbirth, by Richard Moskowitz. Berkeley: North Atlantic, 1992.

The Organon

There are many books on the subject of homeopathy, but only one Organon. It was written by Samuel Hahnemann himself and is a record of his own work as a homeopath. Therefore it is considered the bible of homeopathy, and is perhaps the single most important book on the subject. Hahnemann rewrote and refined his Organon over the years of his practice, so there are now six editions of the work available. The sixth edition contains the discoveries and refinements that Hahnemann made to his practice in the final years of his life and it is recommended reading.

As *The Organon of the Medical Art* was written in German, English editions are only as good as their translations and the quality differs wildly. So choose carefully when you choose your copy of the *Organon*.

The Organon of the Medical Art, by Samuel Hahnemann. Edited and annotated by Wenda Brewster O'Reilly, PhD. Translated by Steven Decker. Birdcage Books, PO Box 2289, Redmond, Washington, 98073-2289, 1997. Because this is a very small company, let me give you the phone number: (206) 285-4737. Simply the best. This is the one translation of the *Organon* that should be on your bookshelf. Nothing else comes close. (I also suggest that you buy the hardback edition, because you will refer to this book again and again over the years.)

The Organon of Medicine, by Samuel Hahnemann. Reprint edition. Translated and with a preface by William Boericke, M.D. New Delhi: B Jain Publishers Ltd,1991. This is the cheapest edition of the *Organon* available today. It is sort of a mongrel edition, with no editor, no apparent guiding hand. But it presents the sixth edition of Hahnemann's work in an adequate translation and is a good, simple edition for the home bookshelf.

Repertories

The repertory is a companion volume to the material medica. Where the material medica lists all remedies alphabetically and then takes them apart individually to list all the symptoms a given remedy can treat, the repertory is instead a list of symptoms. The body is taken from top to bottom: all individual organs and systems are considered, and all possible symptoms associated with those organs and systems are explored. Everything from rashes to the deepest aches and pains is included in this single volume. And again, as each repertory is the work of a single physician, it is important to explore several and to find the one (or two or three) that is right for you.

Repertory of the Homeopathic Materia Medica With Word Index, by J. T. Kent. Reprint edition. New Delhi: B. Jain Publishers, 1986. This is the classic, basic repertory written by American homeopath James Tyler Kent. It belongs on the bookshelf of every student of homeopathy. It is very complete, very basic. Every other homeopath since Kent has based his Repertory on this pioneering work.

Homeopathic Medical Repertory, A Modern Alphabetical Repertory, by Robin Murphy, N.D. Hahnemann Academy of North America, 60 Talisman Drive, Suite 4028, Pagosa Springs, Colorado, 1993. I really like this particular repertory, as it is organized in alphabetical order (many others, including Kent's, operate from the top of the head to the bottom of the feet, making it difficult at times to find the listings for the part of the body you are researching). As a modern repertory, it also has rubrics for conditions and situations that were unknown two hundred years ago.

Synthesis Repertorium, by F. Schroyens. London: Homeopathic Book Publishers, 1993. The Synthesis, as it is known, is one of the most commonly used repertories today. As the name implies, this work pulls together symptoms rubrics from several sources, making it the largest, if not the most complete repertory published in a single volume. Because of the cost of this work, as well as its complexity, this repertory is most often found in the office of medical professionals and not on the home bookshelf.

The Complete Repertory, by Roger Van Zandvoort. 3 volumes. Leidschendam, the Netherlands: IRHIS, 1994. It certainly lives up to its name. Very complete. Very detailed. I personally believe that it could be a bit more user-friendly in its format, but it delivers an extraordinary amount of information.

Materia Medicas

While beginning students of homeopathy can make-do with the lists of remedies and their uses in home guides, more serious students of homeopathy will soon find that they need a material medica of their own. Materia medicas list all remedies in a dictionary format, giving the full range of symptoms associated with a remedy. Without the material medica, a proper drug diagnosis cannot be made. Students would do well to own more than one, as they differ depending upon the experience of the individual practitioner and author. Finding the material medica that's right for you, that reflects your own beliefs of the best possible homeopathic treatment, will be a milestone in the life of any serious student. And that book will be the single most valuable volume in your homeopathic library.

Among the best materia medicas are:

Pocket Manual of Homeopathic Materia Medica, by William Boericke, M.D.

Reprint edition. New Delhi: B. Jain Publishers, 1996. It may seem to be a case of damning something with faint praise, but this volume is in so many homes because it is the cheapest of all the materia medicas. It is far from the most complete, but it is a basic, helpful book. It should be further noted that when Boericke's materia medica was first published it was not particularly well thought of, but it has become the basic and omnipresent materia medica of the modern age. Worth owning, but serious students should not only own this one.

Concordant Materia Medica, by Frans Vermeulen. Haarlem, The Netherlands: Merlijn Publishers, 1994. This is probably the materia medica that I use most often, in that it combines the notes of classical homeopaths Boericke, Phatak, Boger, Lippe, Allen, Pulford, Cowperthwaite, Kent, and Clarke, with Vermeulen's own observations into a wonderful single volume materia medica of astounding richness and depth. I highly recommend this book.

Lotus Materia Medica by Robin Murphy, ND. Lotus Star Academy, 538 Village Drive, Suite 4028, Pagosa Springs, Colorado, 1995. This was created as a companion volume to Murphy's excellent Repertory. (Note that the name of this publishing company has undergone a change, while the address remains the same.) While the materia medica is riddled with typographical errors and some issues of clarity that may have been corrected in future editions, his unique take on the remedies and their uses makes this a solid addition to any homeopathic research library.

Desktop Guide to Keynotes and Confirmatory Symptoms, by Roger Morrison, MD. Hahnemann Clinic Publishing, 828 San Pablo Avenue, Albany, California, 94706, 1993. I really like this book and find it of value again and again. This is a modern materia medica and a bit different from the others. It is not meant to be an exhaustive listing of all remedies and listings. Instead it is a practical look at the remedies that are most commonly used and the guiding symptoms of each.

The Guiding Symptoms of Our Materia Medica, by Constantine Hering, M.D. 10 volumes. Reprint edition. New Delhi: B Jain Publishers, 1997. If you want the complete materia medica, you might want to spring for this one. It takes Hering ten volumes to work his way through the complete list of homeopathic remedies, but this reference work is excellent and well worth the investment.

Systematic Materia Medica of Homeopathic Remedies with Totality of Characteristic Symptoms and Various Indications of Each Remedy, by K.N. Mathur. New Delhi: B Jain Publishers, 1988. This book may be difficult for you to get, but it is well worth the effort. Not a complete materia medica, but a book dedicated to the study of the most commonly used homeopathic remedies. Because of Mathur's unique take on the remedies—one steeped in homeopathy as it is practiced in India—I often turn to this volume when studying the remedies.

Materia Medica Pura, by Samuel Hahnemann. 2 volumes. Reprint edition. New

Delhi: B Jain Publishers, 1986. What was, in its time, the first homeopathic materia medica is, today, far from the best. The book contains Hahnemann's notes on some sixty-odd remedies, ranging from polycrests such as Sulphur and Lycopodium to odd remedies that have been lost in the two hundred plus years of homeopathic practice. I find the book to be of little value in understanding or using the remedies. It is, however, of unique historic interest.

Drug Pictures, by Margaret Tyler. Saffron Walden, England: C. W. Daniel, 1952. This volume is a rather delightful trip into the mind of British homeopath Margaret Tyler. As sort of a combination of a materia medica and a personal memoir, it is a unique volume and one that is not only very interesting to read, but also extremely educational in its content. This book is highly recommended.

Lectures on Homeopathic Materia Medica, by James Tyler Kent. Reprint edition. New Delhi: B Jain Publishers, 1986. It is sort of cheating to list this book in this category, because it is not a true materia medica. Sadly, Kent never wrote one. Instead, the lectures that he gave his students on the various homeopathic remedies have been grouped together in this volume. While it is not the sort of book that you can quickly use to confirm a symptom, it is a valuable study of many of our most-used remedies.

Internet Sites & Resources

www.Homeopathyhome.com: Without a doubt, this is the single best and most comprehensive site on the Internet on the subject of homeopathy. From here, you can link to virtually every other site and research the topic of homeopathy from A to Z. Everything is well organized and laid out, making this site very user-friendly. Further, you can download any number of books and articles about homeopathy from this site, even a free copy of the *Organon*.

www.Homeopathic.org: This is the homepage of the National Center for Homeopathy, one of our nation's largest homeopathic organizations. In addition to information specific to the organization, this site is very helpful for locating homeopathic practitioners across the United States.

www.holisticmed.com/www/homeopathy.html: Use this address to find links to just about anything you can think of pertaining to homeopathy that has an online presence. International links to study groups, organizations, schools, pharmacies, and more are well organized and up to date. Bookmark this site for regular use.

**Finally, come visit me at my own website.
From there you can link to my blog and other places.
You can find me online at www.vintonmccabe.com**

Index

OTHER BOOKS BY VINTON MCCABE

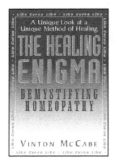

THE HEALING ENIGMA DEMYSTIFYING HOMEOPATHY

In *The Healing Enigma: Demystifying Homeopathy,* McCabe makes use of his full experience of homeopathy to give a fully rounded assessment of the principles of homeopathy and the manner in which it is practiced today. Where other books on the subject are limited in their scope to readers who are interested in the mechanics of its practice, *The Healing Enigma* speaks as much to the practitioners and patients of traditional "allopathic" medicine as it does to those already in the alternative camp.

THE HEALING BOUQUET
EXPLORING BACH FLOWER REMEDIES

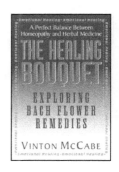

In this volume, McCabe places the Bach Flower Remedies within their natural context—that of homeopathic medicine. In *The Healing Bouquet,* McCabe explores the history of the Bach remedies, as well as the philosophy behind their appropriate use. He gives in-depth portraits of the guiding symptoms for each of Bach's 38 remedies, portraits of emotions and behaviors that will allow readers to identify themselves within these pages.

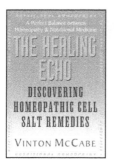

THE HEALING ECHO
DISCOVERING HOMEOPATHIC CELL SALT REMEDIES

In *The Healing Echo,* McCabe offers readers the fundamentals of this simplified form of homeopathic treatment. Further, he gives a comprehensive look at the cell salt remedies themselves, their uses in the treatment of specific conditions, and the manner in which they may become a part of a daily program of nutrition in the home.

HOUSEHOLD HOMEOPATHY A Safe and Effective Approach to Wellness for the Whole Family

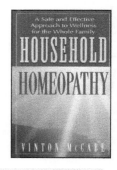

This book makes the subject of homeopathy as down to earth and as practical as it can be. It discusses the most common remedies and how they can be used safely and effectively. *Household Homeopathy* teaches readers how to promote healing in themselves and their loved ones—in their own homes. It covers how to handle remedies, select them, and use them wisely.

Visit www.basichealthpub.com to see all our fine titles.